Fat Scorching Smoothies:

12-Hour Fat Burning Smoothies

19 "Feel Full" Super Smoothies that burn fat for up to 12 hours

(Comes with a bonus 30 Day Email Training Course)

Contents

Introduction..1

Why I Started "Smoothing"...1

Why did I start using a smoothie routine?.........................2

Two Common "Smoothie Routine" Mistakes Easily Fixed..................4

Making Smoothies that are just all Fruit............................4

Repeating a Few Smoothie Recipes...................................5

Getting the Most Out of Every Drop 6

Easily Maximizing Fat Burning Qualities of Smoothies.........6

Sticking to Your Smoothie Routine....................................7

Fat Burning Smoothie Recipes 9

Early Alarm Apple Smoothie...9

Oatmeal Fruit Smoothie 10

Chia Power Up 11

Oatmeal Fruit Smoothie 12

Peach Avocado Smoothie..13

Breakfast of Celebrities 14

Morning Metabolism Explosion 15

Sweet Spinach Slimmer...16

Vegan Delight..17

Peach and White Bean Smoothie 18

Hangover Bloated Belly Blaster 19

Mixed Berry-Cashew Smoothie..20

Amazon Kindle Bonus: 30-in-30 Email Course.......................21

High-Calorie Fat Torching Smoothie Recipes 22

High-Calorie Fat Torching Smoothie #1: Blueberry Greek Yogurt Smoothie.......22

High-Calorie Fat Torching Smoothie #2: Mango Avocado Green Tea Smoothie 23

High-Calorie Fat Torching Smoothie #3: Avacado – Coconut Oil Smoothie 24

High-Calorie Fat Torching Smoothie #4: Berry Banana Smoothie......................25

Mega Full, Fat Melting Recipes 26

#1: Coconut, Cacao, and Green Super Food Smoothie 26

#2: Chia, Banana, Hemp, Kale Super Smoothie...............................27

#3: Super Food Explosion..28

#4: Tropical "Super Food" Smoothie 29

Rules for Making Your Own Recipes 30

12 Best Weight Loss Ingredients 30

6 Ingredients You Want to Avoid in Your Smoothies 33

8 Powerful Fat Burning Super Heroes to Amp
Your Smoothie Benefits 35

Disclaimer 37

Introduction

Fruit smoothies are a fantastic breakfast or meal replacement, but only if you include essential fats and proteins that your body craves. And the proper nutrients and minerals your body needs to actually absorb those fats and proteins. Otherwise your left with that almost "starving" feeling a couple hours later and you'd almost consider kicking a kitten for a Klondike bar.

Don't kick kittens... they're precious.

And don't deprive your body of what it needs, it's precious too.

With precious kittens and the occasional Klondike's in mind, getting on a good, healthy smoothie routine is one of the best ways that I've ever burned off my unwanted fat, helping me hit my big goals.

Why I Started "Smoothing"

Those 'big goals' are personal, but I feel like they're worth sharing because they're what drove me.

The three simple but "big" things that I wanted to accomplish more than anything else were:

1. **To enjoy the sensation of my husband kissing my neck again.** Every single time he'd walk up behind me, wrap his arms around me in a hug, and kiss me on my neck... I just felt fat. He was doing nothing wrong but it started to drive me crazy. And I wasn't about to take it out on him.

2. **To burn my "fat jeans".** I literally wanted to burn them in a fire. I was so sick of only being able to wear that one damn pair of jeans because somehow they were the only ones I could manage to squeeze myself into. They had started to get worn out and tired. And I knew that if I started buying more jeans that were bigger, it'd be game over for me.

3. **To feel 'okay' in my bikini.** We love boating with our friends and family during the summers, we do it every year. When I was at my biggest, I would keep a summer skirt on all day on the boat, except for when I'd take a swim. I just didn't like everyone, or anyone, seeing me like that. I'm sure no one ever would have ever thought anything… but you know how it is, my self-perception was just killing me. I wanted to be able to wear my bikini on a hot summer boating day and not feel mortified.

Where did I need to lose my fat? Just about everywhere. My neck, of course, my arms, my stomach (3 kids changes you forever), and my butt.

Like I said, just about everywhere.

Why did I start using a smoothie routine?

Honestly because I was having a hard time stomaching down all the vitamins, supplements, and "minerals" that I'd mapped out for myself after signing up for weight loss program.

The weight loss program was great. It completely sucked while going through it but it got the weight off.

The issue I had was being able to take all the different pills I needed to be taking daily and not get a "sick" feeling from taking so many.

I was taking about 12 different kinds of vitamins and supplements daily. Sometimes 2-3 pills of some of those supplements.

Getting the vitamins and supplements in liquid form and mixing them into my "feel full" smoothies is what made a HUGE difference for me. I finally started getting consistent, feeling like I had more energy, started seeing results faster (skinnier neck!), felt great about actually following the program, and getting all my needed nutrition.

It's amazing how just getting the main nutrients, like protein, fats, and healthy carbs isn't enough. There's minerals and vitamins you need for actually being able to digest the main nutrients.

(One of the BIG reasons why us girls work our butts off on programs but don't get the results we want – it's often time a digestion block or something else that's happening. I'll get to all this later on.)

So anyways, that's the short version of my story and what started the journey towards me writing this book.

Whatever your goals are and for whatever reason you're hunting for fat burning smoothie recipes – keep at it and don't stop until you get exactly everything you want!

And since what I'm about to share with you in this book worked for me and my close girlfriends, I know there's a really good chance it will help you too.

Two Common "Smoothie Routine" Mistakes Easily Fixed

Making Smoothies that are just all Fruit

This will create a massive spike in your blood sugar that will leave you "crashing" within 3-4 hours. You'll feel like the energizer bunny for the first 90 minutes to 2 hours, but then the slippery slope to the dark side begins.

You'll then get hit with cravings so strong that just the sight of a mini-bag of chips at the gas station will make you start salivating like a feral barn cat.

You can take that only so many times before it's just game over.

It has nothing to do with wanting to lose weight bad enough. That's a bunch of crock.

If just wanting it bad enough was all it took, we'd all look like a magazine cover model that'd make guys trip over their you-know-what's.

Will power and self-discipline in the face of overwhelming biological alarm – which is exactly what your body does when you start to make big changes, going into alarm – shrink to almost nothing.

It's not laziness. It's not weakness.

It's simply how we're wired.

So making smoothies that have lots of healthy fats and proteins in them leaves you feeling full. Feeling full puts the odds in your favor that you'll stick to your plan.

Repeating a Few Smoothie Recipes

Always making the same 2-3 smoothie recipes, over and over and over again. There's many reasons why prison is depressing, one of them being that you always eat the same thing repeatedly.

Yes, it's true that sticking to repeating the same foods in your diet can lead to health improvements. But you've got to at least mix n' match creatively. With all the ingredients available to us, it is possible… so why not help tilt the odds a bit in our favor?

Loading up on nothing but a "greens smoothie" with a farm field full of spinach per smoothie is simply just not going to work.

By your umpteenth time of downing the same thing that week, even food you never thought was that yummy before suddenly starts to look like heavenly deliciousness.

Don't do that to yourself.

That's why I've included 19 recipes in here. Plus later in the book I set you up with rules and main ingredients for experimenting with your own smoothie concoctions.

A smoothie routine should be, and now I know can be, a delicious adventure and experience.

Getting the Most Out of Every Drop

Easily Maximizing Fat Burning Qualities of Smoothies

Doing a minimum effective dose (MED) of movement or exercise right before drinking your smoothie, or before eating any meal for that matter, to the point that you trigger a metabolic demand in your insulin (body gets hungry for food or nutrition) will jumpstart your fat burning 'burners'.

What's the minimum effective dose?

Surprisingly enough, pretty light.

Just 40 wall pushups and 40 squats will trigger enough of a full body metabolic spike that you will maximize how much of your smoothie your burn (instead of storing by converting into fat) and therefore keep the burning going.

A wall pushups is done by simply leaning against a wall at slight angle with your hands on the wall and doing a "push away" from the wall. Modify the angle depending on your strength and ability.

As for the squats, that's just a regular squat down / squat back up movement.

For me, the most effective time to do this was in the bathroom right before my morning shower. So that if I broke a sweat, I'd be showering right away. And then I'd make my smoothie and drink it right after my shower.

You can do a quick spike in your metabolism before any meal to maximize how much of that meal you burn instead of not burning it all and storing some of it.

Sticking to Your Smoothie Routine

So when I started my smoothie routine I wasn't the greatest at sticking to it. And it would be more than a few mornings a week that I'd end up grabbing a spinach feta breakfast wrap at the Starbucks drive thru.

I ended up reading a book that shared strategies for building habits and small things that can set you up for success.

Well one little thing I read and tried made a huge difference in me sticking to my smoothie routine. And anything else I tried after that.

To help me stick with it, I started laying out the ingredients the night before. Pretty simple right?

It's SOOO much easier to lay everything out when you're motivated in the evening rather than in the early morning when you're groggy, maybe have kids to deal with like me, and maybe even in a hurry.

Maybe you can relate to this... I'm always so motivated in the evenings, after looking at one 'motivational' picture after another on Pinterest. Reading a couple blogs I follow. And maybe watching a health & fitness TV show or a few YouTube videos.

Laying out all the ingredients right then and there, in Tupperware, and putting them in the fridge to be ready for me the next morning for some reason just eliminated most of the mental resistance I had to sticking to it.

I'd even put the blender on the counter, front and center.

It sounds simple and small, but trust me if you try this you'll understand exactly what I'm talking about.

Just another tidbit to add...

When I finally got to the point of going for a quick jog every morning, it only happened when I would lay out every single thing I would wear and use the next morning.

My shorts, underwear, socks, shoes, shirt, iPod, glass of water to take my supplements with, the supplements themselves, and my baseball cap.

It was literally all sitting on the counter in my kitchen.

The key is to NEVER have to THINK about it. But just do it.

What I was doing then is *turning it into muscle memory*.

What it does is create a routine. Like showering, brushing your teeth, cleaning your face, and making your hair. Routines *pull* us. We don't even have to think about that morning routine of wash, brush, and comb.

Well, instead of trying to 'discipline' and 'will power' my way through it… I found that simply setting things up the night before for 'no friction or thinking' required the next morning made a massive difference.

Fat Burning Smoothie Recipes

Early Alarm Apple Smoothie

Servings: 1

The ground flaxseed in this recipe definitely leaves you feeling full, while the apple and cinnamon do the trick of jump starting your metabolism. You'll be melting pounds through lunch and into the end of the day. The extra fiber will help cleanse you and you can try making this smoothie the night before, storing it in the fridge, and having it a bit thicker the next day. Whatever you like.

Ingredients:

- 8 ounces coconut water

- 4 raw almonds

- 1 teaspoon vanilla extract

- 1 teaspoon ground cinnamon

- 1 cup chopped apple (about 1 medium apple)

- 1/2 scoop unsweetened protein powder

- 1 tablespoon flaxseed meal (ground flaxseed)

Instructions:

After throwing everything together into your blender, pulse 'em for about 15 seconds. Add three ice cubes if you're going to drink it straight away.

Oatmeal Fruit Smoothie

Servings: 1

The ground up oatmeal will thicken up the smoothie and give it that "full" feeling that'll keep you going into lunch without the usual fruit sugar crash.

Ingredients:

- ¼ cup dry steel oats

- 1 cup frozen fruits, like strawberries, pineapple, or mixed berries

- ½ cup of ice cubes

- 1 packet of stevia

- Ground cinnamon, to taste

Instructions:

First you'll drop the oats in the blender and pulse those bad boys until they get to a powdery consistency. Next just turn off the blender, add 1 cup of water, throw in the rest of the ingredients, and blend it all looks smooth. Enjoy!

Chia Power Up

Servings: 1

Chia seeds are one heck of power food. Not only are they packed with antioxidants, but they also come jam packed with fiber and protein which will keep you feeling full. The protein in this recipe will help curb your sweet tooth cravings for sweet carbs as well!

Ingredients:

- 1 cup frozen mixed berries

- 1/2 cup unsweetened pomegranate juice

- 1/2 cup water

- 1/2 tablespoon chia seeds

Instructions:

Combine all your ingredients into your blender, fire it up, and blend it up. Then pour and enjoy. Feel free to sprinkle some extra chia seeds on top of your glass if you'd like a little extra kick of fiber and "feeling full" effect.

Oatmeal Fruit Smoothie

Servings: 1

The ground up oatmeal will thicken up the smoothie and give it that "full" feeling that'll keep you going into lunch without the usual fruit sugar crash.

Ingredients:

- ¼ cup dry steel oats
- 1 cup frozen fruits, like strawberries, pineapple, or mixed berries
- ½ cup of ice cubes
- 1 packet of stevia
- Ground cinnamon, to taste

Instructions:

First you'll drop the oats in the blender and pulse those bad boys until they get to a powdery consistency. Next just turn off the blender, add 1 cup of water, throw in the rest of the ingredients, and blend it all looks smooth. Enjoy!

Peach Avocado Smoothie

Servings: 1

Yet another very often smoothie recipe overlooked protein and healthy fats super hero… the avocado. You'll be surprised at refreshing taste and sweetness.

Ingredients:

- ¾ cup of unsweetened coconut milk
- 1 cup of frozen peaches
- ¼ cup of avocado

Instructions:

First step is to pour the milk in the blender, then simple add the peaches and the avocado. Next, blend away, and enjoy!

Breakfast of Celebrities

Servings: 1

This is another one from a celebrity trainer favorite… delicious and nutritious, while keeping you feeling full and satisfied for hours. Add this recipe into your smoothie rotation for yummy variety and a healthy pick me up or early morning jump start!

Ingredients:

- 5 raw almonds
- 1 red apple
- 1 banana
- 3/4 cup nonfat Greek yogurt
- 1/2 cup nonfat milk
- 1/4 teaspoon cinnamon

Instructions:

Combine all your ingredients into your blender, fire it up, and blend it up. Then pour and enjoy. If I were you, I'd chop up my apples and almonds into chunks unless you've got one of those blenders that'll whip up a iPhone into a puree.

Morning Metabolism Explosion

Servings: 1

Jump start your metabolism in the morning with this fat-torching smoothie. It's packed with nutrients from ingredients including calcium-rich Greek yogurt, high-fiber strawberries, broccoli, almonds, and spicy cinnamon.

Ingredients:

- 6 ounces vanilla nonfat Greek yogurt

- 10 almonds

- ¼ cup broccoli florets, stems cut off

- 1 cup frozen strawberries

- ¼ cup cannellini beans

- ¾ cup iced green tea

- 1 teaspoon flaxmeal

- ¼ teaspoon cinnamon

Instructions:

Throw all the ingredients into your blender and blend away until smooth. Once you've poured it into your glass, sprinkle a pinch of cinnamon on top and enjoy!

Sweet Spinach Slimmer

Servings: 1

From celebrity trainer and body sculptor Harley Pasternak, this smoothie has been engineered to provide a perfect blend of protein, fiber, and calcium. It's a favorite with celebrities looking to melt extra pounds for a new movie role - and this filling, fat-burning green smoothie will soon be a favorite of yours as well.

Ingredients:

- 2 cups spinach leaves, packed

- 1 ripe pear, peeled, cored, and chopped

- 15 green or red grapes

- 6 ounces fat-free plain Greek yogurt

- 2 tablespoons chopped avocado

- 1 or 2 tablespoons fresh lime juice

Instructions:

Combine all your ingredients into your blender, fire it up, and blend it up. Then pour and enjoy.

Vegan Delight

Servings: 1

Reading the ingredients might make you feel like this is a smoothie for your 'cheat day' (wink!). But coming jam packed with protein, this vegan vanilla milkshake is one of the highest fat burning breakfast smoothies on this list!

Ingredients:

- 1/2 cup soft tofu

- 1 cup vanilla soy milk

- 1 frozen banana

- 1/2 tablespoon peanut butter

Instructions:

Combine all your ingredients into your blender, fire it up, and blend it up. Then pour and enjoy.

Peach and White Bean Smoothie

Servings: 1

This is a great way to spike the protein in your shake, which will jump start your metabolism on burning fat.

Ingredients:

- ½ cup of unsweetened rice milk

- 1 cup of frozen sliced peaches

- ¼ cup canned white beans

- 1/8 teaspoon cinnamon

- Pinch of nutmeg

Instructions:

First you'll need to pour the rice milk into the blender. Next add in all the other ingredients. And finish up by blending it all together. Enjoy!

Hangover Bloated Belly Blaster

Servings: 1

In just a few minutes, you can start burning off fat while also reversing the effects of last night's cocktails that have left you a feeling a bit "bloated". This smoothie will make quick work of the post booze puffiness and also help jump start your energy batteries. You'll be heading out the door with a zing!

Ingredients:

- 3 ounces vanilla nonfat Greek yogurt

- 1 tablespoon almond butter

- 1/2 cup frozen blueberries

- 1/2 cup frozen pineapple

- 1 cup kale

- 3/4 cup water

Instructions:

Combine all your ingredients into your blender, fire it up, and blend it up. Then pour and enjoy.

Mixed Berry-Cashew Smoothie

Servings: 1

It might not be obvious since they're thought a hard nut, but cashews are actually one of the most overlooked smoothie add ins. Raw cashews are the key here, and they're naturally soft and creamy.

Ingredients:

- ¼ cup of raw cashews
- ½ cup of almond milk
- 1 cup of frozen mixed berries

Instructions:

The first step is to put the raw cashews in the blender and grind those little fellas until they're powdered. Add the milk & berries to the party, blend away, and enjoy!

Amazon Kindle Bonus: 30-in-30 Email Course

Amazon Kindle Bonus: 30-in-30 Email Course

Visit the link below to register for your FREE 30 Day Email Course.

http://goo.gl/17NO8A

You'll get 30 emails in 30 days with Step-by-Step instructions for losing weight faster, shortcuts to burning more fat, quick fixes for low energy levels, and easy do-it-yourself skin rejuvenation.

All in bite sized emails of only 500-1200 words!

High-Calorie Fat Torching Smoothie Recipes

Low calorie breakfasts are the devil. When you wake up is exactly when you need a hit of healthy calories. Your metabolism is like a car engine that only starts if it feels you pouring gas into the tank (or exercising). Well, for these smoothies we're looking for fat burning effects even if we're not able to exercise.

So the more healthy and high calorie of a breakfast you can have, the better.

The morning is when your body's metabolism is programmed to burn at its peak, if you get it started properly.

High-Calorie Fat Torching Smoothie #1: Blueberry Greek Yogurt Smoothie

Servings: 1

Ingredients:

- 1/2 cup water

- 1/2 cup fresh or frozen blueberries

- 3/4 cup of plain, Greek yogurt (preferably full-fat)

- 1 tablespoon chia seeds or chia seed gel

- 1/4 teaspoon cinnamon

- 1/2 tablespoon honey (optionally use stevia or maple syrup or 1/2 banana to sweeten)

Instructions:

Combine all your ingredients into your blender, fire it up, and blend it up. Then pour and enjoy.

High-Calorie Fat Torching Smoothie #2: Mango Avocado Green Tea Smoothie

<u>**Servings: 1**</u>

<u>**Ingredients:**</u>

- 1 cup green tea

- 1 cup fresh or frozen mango chunks

- 1/2 medium avocado

- 1 cup spinach

- 1/2 tablespoon coconut oil

- A dash of sea salt

- A little honey, maple syrup, or stevia to sweeten (optional, mango provides enough sweet for me)

<u>**Instructions:**</u>

Combine all your ingredients into your blender, fire it up, and blend it up. Then pour and enjoy.

High-Calorie Fat Torching Smoothie #3: Avacado – Coconut Oil Smoothie

Servings: 1

Ingredients:

- 1 cup water

- 1/2 medium avocado

- 1/2 cup fresh or frozen blueberries

- 1 tablespoon chia seeds or chia seed gel

- 1/2 tablespoon coconut oil (increase to 1 tablespoon over the course of a week)

- 1/4 teaspoon cinnamon

- 1/2 tablespoon honey (optionally use stevia or maple syrup or 1/2 banana to sweeten)

Instructions:

Combine all your ingredients into your blender, fire it up, and blend it up. Then pour and enjoy

High-Calorie Fat Torching Smoothie #4: Berry Banana Smoothie

<u>**Servings: 1**</u>

<u>**Ingredients:**</u>

- 1 cup water

- 1 cup fresh or frozen mixed berries

- 1/2 fresh or frozen banana

- 1 cup spinach

- 1 tablespoon coconut oil

- 1/4 teaspoon cayenne pepper

- 1 tablespoon gelatin (optional, for protein)

<u>**Instructions:**</u>

Combine all your ingredients into your blender, fire it up, and blend it up. Then pour and enjoy.

Mega Full, Fat Melting Recipes

#1: Coconut, Cacao, and Green Super Food Smoothie

This smoothie is packed with fiber, protein, healthy fats, and antioxidants. You'll get a whopping dose of "nutritious and delicious" and metabolism fat burning giddy up!

<u>**Servings: 1**</u>

<u>**Ingredients:**</u>

- 1 cup raw almond milk

- 1 frozen organic banana

- 1 tablespoon raw cacao

- 1 tablespoon raw almond butter

- 1 tablespoon raw expeller-pressed coconut oil

- 1 tablespoon chia, hemp, or flax seeds

- 1 tablespoon maca powder

- 1 tablespoon Vitamineral Green or spirulina

<u>**Instructions:**</u>

Combine all your ingredients into your blender, fire it up, and blend it up. Then pour and enjoy.

#2: Chia, Banana, Hemp, Kale Super Smoothie

Voted the most unique recipe by our writing staff, this smoothie hits you with fiber, protein, and antioxidants from the first gulp to the last slurp.

Servings: 1

Ingredients:

- 3/4 cup unsweetened vanilla almond milk
- 1 pitted date
- 1 tbsp raw shelled hemp seeds (or seeds of your choice)
- 1/2 ripe medium banana
- 1/2 tbsp chia seeds
- 3/4 cup baby kale (or spinach)
- 1 cup ice

Instructions:

Combine all your ingredients into your blender, fire it up, and blend it up. Then pour and enjoy.

#3: Super Food Explosion

This is a very "feeling full" smoothie that will leave you feeling like you actually just ate a full meal. It's chock full of protein, calcium, potassium, healthy fats, and iron.

Servings: 1

Ingredients:

- 1 cup raw almond milk

- 2 frozen organic bananas

- 1 cup organic baby spinach

- ¼ cup raw almonds, soaked

- ¼ cup goji berries (3 to 4 reserved for garnish)

- 1 tablespoon raw cashew butter

- 1 teaspoon raw coconut shreds (for garnish)

- 1 teaspoon organic raw cacao nibs (for garnish)

- 1 teaspoon raw Brazil nuts, ground fine (for garnish)

Instructions:

Combine all your ingredients into your blender except for the garnishes. Blend things up and pour into your glass. Then add the coconut, Brazil nuts, goji berries, and cacao nibs on top. Enjoy!

#4: Tropical "Super Food" Smoothie

This delicious smoothie is jam packed with tropical flavors and antioxidants. The fruits, coconut milk, and maca powder combine to give the taste of a sun kissed tropical beach while leaving you feeling full and ready to go.

Servings: 1

Ingredients:

- 1 cup raw coconut milk (or a little more to achieve desired consistency)
- 1 frozen organic banana
- ¼ cup papaya, cubed and frozen
- ¼ cup mango, cubed and frozen
- ¼ cup pineapple, cubed and frozen
- 1 teaspoon maca powder
- 1 teaspoon goji berry powder
- 1 teaspoon bee pollen
- Slice fruit of choice for garnish

Instructions:

Combine all your ingredients into your blender, fire it up, and blend it up. Then pour and enjoy.

Rules for Making Your Own Recipes

12 Best Weight Loss Ingredients

Coconut oil: As you read earlier, low calorie breakfasts are the devil. And coconut oil is the star player in nipping that problem in the bud. Providing plenty of healthy fat for keeping you full and jump starting your metabolism (only beaten in jump starting powers by jumper cables direct to the nipples). Make sure you get it extra virgin, in a glass jar only.

Tea/water/ice: Try to usually replace recipe calls for milk or fruit juice with tea, water, or ice. Green tea specifically helps to burn fat and jump start the metabolism. You can also use herbal fruity teas to give your recipe a little more sweetness without using sugar coma inducing fruit juices.

Healthy fats: Our bodies are kind of funny… whatever we put into them often is what they begin to crave and burn more of. So go figure that eating fats (healthy fats) will get you craving more fats and in turn end up triggering your body to burn more of the fat you've already stored. Brand this inside your eye lids: you cannot lose weight or burn fat without consuming plenty of healthy fats. You can get healthy fats into your smoothies with avocados, nut butters, nuts, and coconut oil.

Cayenne pepper: Spicy things spike your weight loss, it doesn't just give you warm burn on the lips… it gets your metabolism burning as well, which is exactly what you want for weight loss and burning fat. As if all that wasn't enough to qualify for the list, research has come out showing that eating cayenne pepper in the morning can curb your cravings for carbs later on in the day.

Pulp from fruit: The pulp is where ALL the fiber in fruits is hanging out. And you want fiber in your smoothies if your smoothies are to be burning fat for 12+ hours! Include it in your smoothies when the recipe calls for fruits, and create recipes that include it.

Berries: Pretty much any berry you can think of is packed with antioxidants for your healthy, brings a punch of fiber to keep you feeling full, and adds heaps of yummy flavor without adding tons of sugary calories. That may be why some think that berries are the ultimate super food.

Greek yogurt: Greek yogurt reigns king among all yogurts in terms of protein. That means it'll do a much better job of jump startinig your metabolism and keep you full. And listen up, get the full fat option… 'diet' or 'fat free' or 'reduced fat' just about anything means "some other kind of poo poo was added". I know, doesn't sound very official, so do your own research if you like.

Chia seeds: This little unsung nutrient hero is a powerful super food for weight loss. They're packed with fiber and protein which is what keeps you feeling full. They're jam packed with nutrients like antioxidants, omega-3 fatty acids, and calcium. But wait, not done yet… they also absorb bad toxins while merrily traveling through you. Not bad, eh?

Leafy greens: High in fiber, high in minerals, and much needed phytonutrients, most smoothies should have at least some greens in them. Spinach, dandelion, kale, and romaine lettuce are just a few good greens to keep on our short list. The key here variety… so that you can maximize health benefits from different types of greens. They're not all exactly the same in nutrition just because they're the same color!

Cinnamon: This is a favorite of Tim Ferriss (see his best-selling book "Four Hour Body") because this lovely spice happens to help regulate blood sugar levels by improving how well you can use and burn glucose. This means your body doesn't store as much excess blood glucose as fat. The kicker is that it happens to work the best on fat deposits stored around your abs!

Avocado: These bad boys are what gives many a smoothie its creaminess while also providing you with the protein and healthy fats you need to trigger weight loss. In addition, they do a wonderful job of leaving you full which is why quite a few of our recipes have them included.

Stevia: This is a natural sweetener that comes from a plant that you can add to your smoothies if you find that they're not quite sweet enough for you.

6 Ingredients You Want to Avoid in Your Smoothies

Fruit juice: The average amount of sugar that a person in the US ingests nowadays compared to even 50 years ago is absolutely ridiculous. Just go do the research for yourself. The overwhelming majority of fruit juices that you'd find on the store shelves are chock full of bad sugars. The fruit juice also doesn't have the fiber nutrients anymore that the original fruit once did. Double whammy.

Protein Powders: Natural sources or protein are the best. In addition, powders that you'd buy at popular fitness and nutrition stores like GNC actually have many hidden sugars in them. It doesn't always say "sugar". Words like aspartame, cane crystals, dextrin, dextrose, evaporated cane juice, xylose, sucrose, and on and on are all just another word for sugar – often time a synthetic form too, which is even worse. Be really careful of the protein powder that you choose to use, if you at all.

Overdoing Sweet Fruit: Again, the naughty culprit sugar raising its naughty head again. Even if you're using natural, fresh fruits… they are a source of sugars. In moderation, fresh fruits are perfect and the staple of most smoothie recipes. But overload on even these healthy, natural sugars and you'll cause spikes in your blood sugar levels. This creates a domino effect of reactions that are not healthy, like digestive problems.

Sweeteners: Again, sugars are simply killing us. Over consumption of sugar is one of the leading causes of accelerated aging, inflammation, fatigue, etc,. – so make sure you are aware of what you're putting into your smoothies… and into your body. Stevia is an okay, natural sweetener. You can also use honey and maple syrup in very sparing moderation. Suggest sticking to just Stevia if you can.

Dairy: Most dairy should be avoided since most sources of dairy are full of additional calories that you don't want.

Exceptions can be made for raw milk and plain full-fat Greek yogurt because they are super high in protein and have very little sugar.

Canned fruits or Vegetables: Turns out that canned fruits and veggies tend to have a lot of additional sugars, preservatives, and salt that spike the amount of calories in them. Which is exactly what you don't want – unhealthy calories. Only use fresh or frozen fruits and veggies. Fresh is the first choice and frozen is the second choice. Frozen fruits and veggies retain their nutrients much longer than the canned option, and they don't have all the added preservatives.

8 Powerful Fat Burning Super Heroes to Amp Your Smoothie Benefits

Honey and Bee Pollen: Honey and bee pollen are to very potent additions to your smoothies. They are a source of vitamins, proteins, and minerals have been used to fight asthma, acne, anemia, indigestion, fatigue, and arthritis. Since both naturally taste sweet, you won't require additional sweetener if you add them to your smoothie recipe.

Aloe Vera: Think we've spent too much time in the sun and added the aloe vera plant to this list by mistake? Think again. This isn't just for soothing sunburns. This magical little plant has a long list of benefits, only some of which include reducing inflammation, stabilizing blood sugar, hydrating with electrolytes, preventing kidney stones, lowering cholesterol, slowing tumor growth, preventing kidney stones, improving digestion, and relieving muscle and joint pain. All you have to do is buy the leaves at your grocery store and cut them open to get the gel inside. The gel is the only part you add to any of your smoothies.

Hemp Seeds: Yes indeed, these seeds do in fact come from the marijuana plant. But don't worry, these seeds no or very little of the compound that produces the 'high' feeling. In addition to having omega-6 and omega-3 fatty acids – hemp seeds also contain "super" fatty acids called gamma-linoleic acid and stearidonic acid. All these healthy fats combine to prevent heart disease, improve brain health, improve immune system functions, and regulate blood sugar.

Goji Berries: As always, the berry family just seems to be full of benefits and nutrition. The Goji berry is one of the healthiest of the berry family, packed with minerals, vitamins, antioxidants, and protein. The list of benefits from the Goji berry include improved vision, protection against heart disease, anti-aging effects, and production of human growth hormone (necessary for anti-aging).

Maca: This little power player originates in the Andes Mountains of Peru and packs a wollop of virility. Originally used by Peruvians to boost virility, it is now known to also lower stress, improve mood, increase sexual function and fertility, and improve energy levels. As if all that wasn't enough to qualify Maca for your smoothie, it happens to be nutrient dense with vitamins C and E, magnesium, calcium, iron, zinc, phosphorus, protein, and B vitamins!

Spirulina: While the Maca is brought to us by the natives of Peru, this power player is brought to us by the Aztecs. This magical ingredient can improve the functioning of your immune system, relieve suffering from autoimmune diseases, block histamine production, relieve allergy symptoms, and sponge out toxins and heavy metals from your body. It is also nutrient dense, packed with omega-6 and omega-3 fatty acids, vitamin K, B vitamins, vitamin E, zinc, beta carotene, iron, copper, and trace minerals.

Cacao: So first off, since it's not processed and therefore still full of its original nutrients, this will be a bitter tasting version of what you normally find sweet and addicting. Get raw cacao and enjoy another long list of benefits including regulating blood sugar, lowering blood pressure, improving brain function, increasing blood flow, improving vision, lowering cholesterol, and improving your vision. The stevia and natural fruits you already have in your smoothie should do the trick of cutting through the bitter taste.

Acai: So far humans have yet to discover any other fruit that contains as much antioxidants as acai. They also happen to be a source of trace minerals, monounsaturated fats, proteins, and fibers... with very few calories to boot. As if that wasn't enough, they'll in killing cancer cells, lowering your cholesterol levels, and helping with anti-aging.

Disclaimer

www.ingramcontent.com/pod-product-compliance
Lightning Source LLC
Chambersburg PA
CBHW070131290526
45789CB00005B/2203